HEALTHY
&
HYDRATED

The Key to Vibrant Living

Inside Out & Outside In

Pamela Roberts CEC CCE CHC

DEDICATION

This book is dedicated to those seeking healthier and happier lifestyles, no matter your age. I challenge you to reach beyond your comfort zone and discover what magic you can achieve.

This book is dedicated to Robert whose support has been never ending as we grow vibrantly old together. Stay healthy and stay hydrated.

Additionally, I dedicate this book to my son Tyler who is embarking on his life after college. It is an exciting time for everyone!

CONTENTS

ACKNOWLEDGMENTS

I would like to acknowledge Fabienne Frederickson and *The Client Attraction Business School* for the challenge to write this book and to get this message out there. The support and encouragement from the tribe of Cabbies has been more than I could have ever imagined.

Deep gratitude also goes out to Robert who showed me that what was obvious to me is the exact message many people need to hear.

FORWARD BY
JOHN CONTI, DMD;
THE NUTRI-DOC

As a practicing dentist of Whole Health and Implant Dentistry for over 26 years I have sadly watched my patients' health decline as the numbers of prescriptions have increased. The information that people need to take control of their own health is fragmented and surrounded by so much fat that even those that are diligent in seeking the simple answers to good health are often misled.

Proper Hydration is the key to life. In many parts of the world the struggle is for clean drinking water. Hydration is an essential part of life. For those trained in ACLS (Advanced Cardiac Life Support), giving fluids thru an IV could save a life.

As critical as hydration is to your health, many people take drinking water for granted and reach for other popular beverages instead. Even at the collegiate and professional sports levels, athletes, who have team doctors, still suffer from dehydration.

This area has become particularly fascinating to me since the athlete and the teams have so much money at stake. Insuring that the athlete is capable of performing at their highest level is vitally important for both, yet often neglected.

For the sports fan, the news of a professional sports star developing Deep Vein Thrombosis (DVT) is heard in the news often. How are high trained, physically fit, professional athletes, developing blood clots?

For the highly trained athlete, dehydration is a major component for blood clot formation. The athlete is in great shape, has low blood pressure, sweats a lot, and often sits stationary on long plane trips. Without proper hydration the athlete's blood becomes thick, the pump pressure is weak, the body isn't moving, and the blood clots form.

Proper hydration is a key component of my "Health Diet" that I preach about. Chef Pamela Roberts perfect blend of knowledge on hydration and food is essential for those determined to become healthier.

This book is a must read for all of those interested in taking charge of their own health Good quality water in your diet provides the foundation for good health. Proper hydration is a solid platform on which you can build upon.

John M. Conti, DMD "The Nutri Doc"

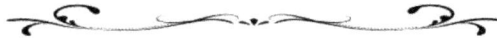

Dr. Conti is a professional speaker giving presentations on whole food, plant based diet and the impact of health.

- Graduate of the University of Florida, College of Dentistry

- (1990 DMD)

- University of Florida Implant Educators Residency (2011-2012)

- Fellow in the International Congress of Oral Implantology

- Restorative and Implant Dental Practice for 23 years

Dr. Conti is an Environmental Scientist with the Southwest Florida Water Management District.

Disclaimer:

If you suffer from heart disease or are under care for your heart for any reason, you will need to consult your doctor for advice and approval to begin a water consumption routine. With many kinds of heart disease, fluids are restricted. Always get your cardiologists approval, if under medical care.

Additionally, if you are taking medications or have any dietary restrictions, ALWAYS consult your doctor and medical care team before starting or changing any current regime you are on. This includes increasing your water intake.

This advice is intended for normal, healthy individuals who live active lifestyles and have no serious medical issues.

This advice is not intended to replace, supersede or discount any medical professional care plan. If you have questions, consult your medical care team for personalized advisement.

1. AN INTRODUCTION TO HYDRATION

A global study by the AC Neilson Company determined that over sixty percent of the population confirms that being in your sixties is the new middle age. This gives true meaning to "sixty is the new forty."

With the baby boomer generation growing older, there are more people over the age of sixty than ever before. The golden years are now being redefined, just as the baby boomer generation has redefined everything it has ever touched, the aging process is being redefined.

Joint replacement is commonplace where a generation ago, a bad hip or knee often meant wheelchair confinement. Now, it is common practice to simply replace bum joints, spend a few weeks in recovery and then resume an active lifestyle.

Being sixty or seventy today looks a lot different today than it did fifty years ago. You do not see as many frail, dwindling older folks with the baby boomer generation. What you do see are people who are leading more active lifestyles, being stronger in older years than others in their thirties and forties.

What is amazing is the perception of age. The perception that growing old is helpless; dependent on others, with loss of mobility and health. With the generation that is entering their golden years now, we are seeing more vibrant, active, self-sufficient and happy people than ever before.

> *Part of active aging is diet and nutrition of which hydration is a key pillar.*

Beyond our basic primary need of quality food and beverage, as humans, we have other basic needs that need to be met.

Just as the body will take water from all other parts of the body to support the basic function of five major organs, humans will overcompensate in other areas to overcome lack or need in another. We need to strive to maintain a balance in all areas for optimum health. Remember the term "being well rounded" when we were growing up? Ideally, our human experience compels us to explore many areas of life. Exploring love and relationship, spirituality, and diet and nutrition leads to deeper understanding and the ability to relate to something you comprehend on a deeper level.

A basic human response to being uncomfortable is to find comfort. We avoid discomfort at all costs. Unfortunately, some people cannot and do not acknowledge the emotions they feel. This can lead to being stuck and distracted. If you notice an area in your life that can use improvement, decide to face it, work on it and make changes if you need to. Deal with what is making you uncomfortable so you can grow past it.

Beyond Maslow's *Hierarchy of Needs* with physiological needs forming the base, the needs for food, water, clothing, and shelter are the most basic and need to be fulfilled first before growth or expansion can happen. We need to feel secure before we can reach out of our boxes. If our boxes need work, then work on them.

Here is a list of some of the basic needs beyond food and water.

In no particular order:

Sleep – sleep deprivation plagues our society. To be at your best and in top form, it is important to get your minimum seven to eight hours of uninterrupted sleep each night. Get up at the same time every day and go to bed the same time if you can. Make getting enough sleep a priority and you will see an improvement in your performance mentally and physically as well as a reduction of stress.

Movement – Use it or lose it. Walk, stand, stretch, dance or do yoga. Use what you want to keep every day. This is especially important as you age. Like to walk? Walk every day to ensure you can as you progress in years.

Sexuality – We have a primal need to connect with a sexual partner, no matter what the age. Sexual energy is powerful. Some celibates claim clearer and more productive lives once they became celibate. There are processes that teach you how to channel sexual energy elsewhere so you can control it rather than it control you. And there are those who lead active, healthy sex lives well into the golden years.

Love – every human and animal and other forms of life all need love to thrive. Once we leave home, if we had a good loving home, we search for it until we find it. If we didn't have a nurturing, loving home, that we try to find one or create one. We all live longer, better lives with someone to share it with whether that be siblings, parents, children or extended family or pets.

Rhythm – Routine and systems help us to believe we are secure and safe. The rhythms of nature, of music and of our tapping feet or snapping fingers; rhythm can make us happy and lifts us higher in our existence plane. Rhythm is not routine and routine is not rhythm. The heart beat is a rhythm, our breathing is a rhythm; our sleep/wake cycle is a rhythm and so is our hunger pattern. Have an irregular heartbeat, interrupt your sleep cycle, go without food, or even get constipated and you will experience quickly how important it is for rhythm to be there.

Connection with Meaning or Purpose – to feel we matter, what we do can make a difference and how we spend our time changes lives. This connects us with our reason for being here, helps us determine our legacy and how to contribute to higher good in the communities we live in. For some, this is obvious from early on, some discover their calling or meaning later in life. Some still, remain unaware such a thing could exist their entire lives. Set goals, be somebody, share your unique gifts with the world. If you do not, every one of us will miss out on your unique gifts. Who else is there to be you but you?

Relaxation – In order for the mind and body to grow, it needs a time of rest. Relaxation of the body and mind is critical to be able to balance hectic modern day lives. Overwhelm is a lack of being able to relax. Relaxation allows the brain to take in all the information it has recently been exposed to. Relaxing gives the brain a chance to process and prepare to receive more. If you don't take time for this, you may find yourself constantly hitting a wall and not making progress. If this is you, take a couple of hours, and afternoon or even a whole day or weekend, whatever it takes to give yourself a break from the overwhelm. When you come back, it won't seem so complicated, you may see solutions you couldn't before and you will find a sudden Ah Ha moment. All because you took a break, gave your brain a rest and let it get ready for more.

Now isn't that a great excuse for a massage?

Food and Drink – seems to be the first of the needs to get satisfied, more than sex. Being hungry is something we all try to satisfy at least three times a day. The body needs both food and drink to function properly.

You can go without food for a couple of weeks but you cannot go without water or fluids for more than three to five days. With our bodies between 60-75% water, does that really surprise you?

Sometimes people will overcompensate in one area of need when lacking in another. An example would be overeating when not in a relationship; or over exercising or not exercising at all when lost for purpose or meaning.

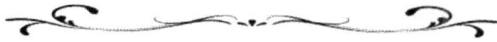

The human body is a complex machine that has many needs. One of the simplest needs is water. This book explains the body's need for water, how the body uses water and why it is beneficial to you to be fully hydrated.

As an educator, I found that once people understand the why of a particular task or program, they are more likely to change or perform certain behaviors than not. If they do not understand why, the chances of anyone performing a desired behavior for any length of time is very low. People need to know what is in it for them and understand why they are spending their time doing as they are.

What is in it for you when you read this book? My intention is for you be motivated enough to review your hydration needs. Then, armed with understanding why, you will make the adjustments to be fully hydrated so you can reap the rewards of vibrant health and an active lifestyle.

The goal of this book is to get you to drink more water and beneficial fluids to enhance your health and ensure a vibrant life through the aging years. There is no need to suffer various health maladies when drinking enough water every day can solve or prevent many problems caused by dehydration.

In this book, you will discover a few recipes for refreshing beverages to get your thinking mind moving on how to create refreshing beverages to replace soda and other sugar and chemical laden drinks. The appendix has several charts and quick reference materials just in case you need to look up some information quickly instead of searching the book for the information later.

How we age is our choice. Genetics play a small role but how we conduct our lives makes all the difference in the world. Health and vibrant living depend upon being properly hydrated. Understand that we are complex beings and we are in total control of how we hydrate our bodies.

I can't stress this enough, because I care about you and want you to have a vibrant healthy life:

If you suffer from heart disease or are under care for your heart for any reason, you will need to consult your doctor for advice and approval to begin a water consumption routine. With many kinds of heart disease, fluids are restricted. Always get your cardiologists approval, if under medical care.

Additionally, if you are taking medications or have any dietary restrictions,

ALWAYS consult your doctor and medical care team before starting or changing any current regime you are on. This includes increasing your water intake.

This advice is intended for normal, healthy individuals who live active lifestyles and have no serious medical issues.

This advice is not intended to replace, supersede or discount any medical professionals care plan. If you have questions, consult your medical care team for personalized advisement.

2. THE IMPORTANCE OF WATER

Three out of four people are chronically dehydrated. Most people don't realize it. Some don't care or see the connection between hydration and health while others are aware and making every effort to hydrate.

Do you suffer from afternoon fatigue? Do you have the occasional mild headache? Trouble focusing on the task at hand? Do you suffer from muscle cramps or dry mouth? Do you have problems digesting your food, have heart burn or are you constipated?

All of these are signs of dehydration and they can all be easily avoided. Gaining and maintaining health through drinking water is the most economical thing you will ever do for your health and you will reap great rewards physically and mentally.

Over half of the weight the average human carries around on its frame is water weight. When you take that into consideration, you begin to understand how important water is to healthy functioning of the body's systems.

According to a University of Washington study, the thirst mechanism is so weak in 37% of the American population that it is often mistaken for hunger.

Do you ever feel lightheaded or weak or perhaps shaky and think you need to get something to eat? "Getting peckish," is what a friend used to call it. Next time that happens, drink a simple eight-ounce glass of water, room temperature, and see how you feel. In most cases, the thirst can satisfy those hunger pangs, yet often, thirst isn't recognized as what is needed.

Lack of water is the number one trigger for daytime fatigue, mild headaches, and constipation. These are the simple, common issues mild dehydration uses to alert you to the need for more water before it gets too late.

Your body will pull water from all areas in order to support five major organs: the brain, heart, lungs, liver and kidneys.

The average American has a body weight percentage between 45-75% depending upon your age, gender and muscle mass.

Babies are born with 75% water weight that adjusts to around 65% within the first year of life.

Water weight percentage will also fluctuate based upon the liquid consumption of the individual and the lifestyle they live. Active, vibrant lives have more water requirements than sedentary lifestyles. Even someone sick, unable to get out of bed, has basic water level requirements. Breathing uses water. Body functions use water.

> *The human body will lose about eight ounces of water during an eight hour sleeping session*

Breathing, sweating, digestion, eye and joint lubrication, skin, regulating body temperatures are some examples of how the body uses water as you sleep.

It makes sense to recommend drinking a glass of water (a mere one- cup) first thing in the morning will help your body regulate systems and start off the day which is better than guzzling two or three cups of coffee which may also be laden with cream and sugar or worse, artificial sweeteners and fake milk-like whiteners.

If you start to think of your body as a living machine that needs proper lubrication and high quality fuel to run properly, you will start to look at water and food consumption differently.

The fine machine that is the human body requires fresh, clean water as a necessary functioning element just as a fine car requires quality oil to function properly.

The Journal of Biological Chemistry published a study by HH Mitchell discussing the various amounts of water in the body's organs.

Blood Plasma – body's total	83 - 90%
Brain	73%
Heart	73%
Lungs	83%
Muscles	79%
Kidneys	79%
Skin	64%
Liver	72%

It is interesting to note that while the skeleton is 30-40% of the total body weight, when the water is removed from the bones, half of that weight is lost.

All life, as we know it, needs water. Water is a sign of life. We look for evidence of water to support the theory of the existence of life. Yet, remarkably, there are a good amount of people who don't drink any water at all. How do they stay alive?

Dr. Alyson Goodman, a medical epidemiologist employed by The Center for Disease Control and Prevention (CDC), conducted a study that revealed nearly one in ten Americans drink no water every day. *None at all!*

Dr. Goodman comments about the study results:

"Mind boggling. Water is vital to life. Many health risks decrease when you drink plain water."

These health risks include kidney stones which are complicated by not drinking enough fluids and Urinary Tract Infections (UTI) are helped by water to flush out the toxins and bad bacteria from the bladder. When toxins remain in the system without water, problems arise like kidney stones and severe infections.

Upon reaching the first conclusion of the experiment, Dr. Goodman couldn't believe the data. So she and her team rechecked yet the conclusions remained the same.

Dr. Goodman deduces these non-water drinkers are getting whatever liquid their body needs to function from coffee, sodas, sugary drinks, alcoholic beverages and various foods they eat. While not the best quality or source, it is fluid the body uses the best it can.

Imagine trying to run a high quality machine on little or no lubricant and on the cheapest fuel.

How long would you expect it to perform well?

How long would you expect it to last?

How long would it be dependable?

If you wouldn't do that to a fine automobile, why would you do it to your own body?

> *"Water is vital to life. Many health risks decrease when you drink plain water."*
>
> Dr. Alyson Goodman, CDC

3. BODY OF WATER

The chemical reactions that take place in the human body require certain amounts of water in order to function properly.

Our circulation, nerves, skin, digestion and lymphatic systems all depend on having water to do the work they do. Without it, everything struggles to do the job as best it can, putting strain and stress on the entire system.

Next, we will briefly discuss the five major organs the body will go to lengths to protect over all other parts of the body.

Your human body really is a remarkable machine.

Always follow your doctor's advice before staring any new regime, even drinking water, especially if you take medications. Ask your doctor if drinking water is right for you. Then ask your doctor how much water they drink every day.

The Brain:

Being between 85% and 95% water, a small drop in hydration will trigger mild headaches, confusion, fuzzy thinking, trouble making clear decisions, and difficulty doing simple math calculations, short term memory loss and an inability to focus.

A drop of 2% of hydration is enough to cause difficulty focusing on a computer screen.

Rather than grab pain killers for that headache, drink twenty ounces of water over the next fifteen minutes. Wait twenty minutes, and then see how you feel. Continue to sip water throughout the day.

Be sure to seek medical attention for headaches and other issues that are severe or are not normal to you.

Never force water on an unconscious or choking person.

The Heart:

The heart pumps the blood all through the body. It's one muscle that never stops working, hopefully. At 73% water, the heart needs water to keep moving smoothly. The blood it pumps, when properly hydrated, is between 83-90% water. When the body is dehydrated, it takes water from the blood to keep the heart moving, making it harder to keep moving the toxins and nutrients through the body as it is designed to do. This result is that everything has to work harder to move and eliminate waste and toxins in a timely manner.

Proper hydration may help reduce the risk of heart disease.

Heart disease treatments often restrict fluids because a diseased heart has a hard time moving fluids around the body. Often heart disease makes the body retain fluid which pools in the legs, ankles and feet, evidenced by swelling in those areas. Restriction of fluids in the case of heart disease is so the heart won't have to work so hard trying to pump all the extra fluids through the body. The heart has a hard time getting the fluids through the body's systems for proper elimination.

The Lungs:

Breathing uses water. At 83-85% water, these marvelous life giving orbs in our chest need water to stay lubricated, to move mucus out of the lungs in a timely manner, and to lubricate the throat and nasal breathing passages.

A drop in hydration will trigger a histamine response which closes capillaries in the lungs in an effort to retain moisture but making it much harder to breathe.

When the mucus membranes are fully hydrated they help protect the body from disease.

The Liver:

The liver filters blood coming from the digestive tract processes some drugs and detoxifies toxins for the body. Without proper hydration, the liver develops issues. Some of the diseases that can happen from chronic dehydration are: fatty liver, hepatitis, and cirrhosis caused by long term damage. These diseases become complicated further when hydration levels fall to lower than 73% the liver needs to function properly.

One function of the liver is to convert fat to energy. Without proper hydration, the liver will assist the kidneys doing their job. This causes the liver to store fat rather than burning fat for energy, as it would with adequate hydration.

The Kidneys:

The kidneys filter waste products out of our bodies. When there is not enough water, and waste products are not completely removed; this can result in kidney stones and other complications. The National Kidney Research Foundation suggests drinking two liters of water per day to reduce the risk of developing kidney stones and to keep the kidneys properly hydrated at 80%.

If you've ever had a kidney stone, you would go to great lengths to never have one again.

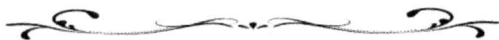

As you may realize, water plays an important role in how our bodies function and perform. As an interconnected group of functioning organs, water plays a major role in the health and proper functioning of these organs.

These five areas are of the utmost importance and the body will protect them in spite of others areas also needing hydration.

So instead of reaching for aspirin or ibuprofen, have a good solid drink of water and then continue to sip water throughout the rest of the day. You will be amazed at how this will solve a simple headache, hunger pangs and afternoon fatigue.

To prove it to yourself, make a note of how you feel, how much water you drank, how much time passed before you felt relief and note how you feel.

While most people don't say "hey, I feel a rush of energy from drinking water" what does happen is one day they realize the pain is gone, the joints move better, the skin fits and you don't get sick as often as you once did. It's hard to notice something that is not there. You will notice that you look and feel better.

Pretty cool stuff from a glass of water.

I had a student, Helen, who claimed the only beverage she ever drank was Southern sweet tea. She drank several 32 ounce cups full each day. By several, I mean four to six of these 32 ounce super sweet cups of tea. In her mid, tea was made with water so she thought she was drinking water.

She could get a free refill from the Circle-K if she brought her cup in with her and so she did. Every day, and every single time she passed a Circle –K.

Here are a couple of things: Tea itself isn't bad for you, neither is the lemon squeeze so common in good iced tea. However, in case you don't know truly deep Southern sweet tea, the elixir is more like tea syrup than a refreshing beverage. Sinfully sweet. It is job security for dentists.

During a nutritional cooking class one day I challenged everyone to drink more water and to keep track of how they felt.

Several months later, Helen came back to me. I hardly recognized her. She had dropped a lot of weight, her skin was vibrant, she had a bounce in her step; she was glowing!

Helen told me that the day I challenged the class to drink water, she thought she would try it as a last resort. Before, Helen had been overweight and suffering from various maladies on a regular basis. Now, after drinking water steadily for six months, she felt like she had a new grip on life. She said once she began drinking the right amount of water, her snacking and nibbling stopped; her meals got better and the pounds fell away. Of course the mere reduction in sugar consumption alone would result in weight loss, but it was so good to see someone who changed their life because they decided to drink more water.

This advice is not meant to replace your doctor's advice or recommendations. If you have any questions at all regarding the consumption of water and the effect on your medications, please consult your medical team for guidance.

These recommendations are meant for healthy individuals with no major medical issues.

4. THE EFFECTS OF DEHYDRATION

In the last chapter we took a quick look at the five major organs the body protects above all else. In this chapter we will look at the effects of dehydration on the rest of the body. Hopefully you will realize how you can prevent dehydration and take steps to ensure your health, a great body and glowing skin.

The muscles contain 75% water. One sign of not enough water is muscle cramping and weakness. Sometimes muscles will twitch and shake or become weak as the body pulls water from the muscles to support the vital organs.

As a chef by trade, whenever we "worked the line" it was important to have water to drink. We used to tell the new kids, "If you're not drinking every five minutes, you're going to be in trouble in ten." And sure enough, some of the new line cook cowboys would be passing out on the line because they were nipping beer or brandy or guzzling Mountain Dew while their bodies were starving for some simple water. We'd simply drag them off the line, toss some ice on them and get back to work. New cooks on the line have so much to learn.

Two-thirds of the water in the body is intracellular fluid; the other third is extracellular fluid. The amount of water varies according to the organ or system.

The cells maintain a specific gradient concentration of sodium inside the cell and serum outside the cell. When excess water is on the outside of the cell, it draws the sodium out of the cell as it tries to maintain the proper concentration of gradient inside and outside the cell. As water accumulates the serum sodium concentration dilutes and drops creating hyponatremia which means too much water is in the system, the sodium balance is off kilter and there's going to be a problem if balance isn't restored quickly.

Osmosis is another way cells attempt to regain electrolyte balance via water outside the cell permeating the membrane and entering the inside of the cell.

Did you know…?

Understanding the concept of osmosis is essential to knowing how to cook meat like a master. If you understand the process you will know when to salt and when to sear meat. The same theory holds true for all cooking but meat is the most susceptible to salting at the wrong time.

Sodium, potassium, chloride, calcium and magnesium are the minerals that make up electrolytes. Electrolytes circulate throughout the body delivering glucose and amino acids both inside and outside the cells.

Each electrolyte is balanced with an equal and opposite electrical charge to manage nutrient and waste flow and many other functions. Water is essential for this to work properly.

Dehydration occurs when the intake of water is less than the amount of water the body uses. In other words you lose more liquid than you take in. This can happen from being extremely active, being in an extreme environment (think heat) or being sick with vomiting and diarrhea are key areas to take steps to prevent dehydration.

What happens if you get dehydrated? How can you tell if you are or not?

The first symptoms of dehydration are dry lips and a dry, sticky mouth. You may notice you are thirsty. This would be a great time to have between ten to twenty ounces of water over the next few minutes. Gradually consume the water; don't guzzle it all at once.

In most cases, people will grab the lip balm and a bite to eat instead of recognizing thirst.

You may get drowsy or feel sleepy. Dehydration is the number one cause of daytime fatigue.

Your skin is dry, especially in the winter months when indoor heat dries out the air. Body lotions don't seem to last, skin is itchy, prone to frequent rashes, flaking and redness. Your skin feels like is doesn't fit your body anymore, making you cranky and irritable.

You feel a slight headache that nags at you; you feel lightheaded and dizzy. You have trouble focusing on what you are doing. As dehydration progresses, you have difficulty making decisions and you become confused and argue easily.

Digestion gives you heartburn and you suffer from constipation. Your mouth is dry, and when you cry there are little or just a few tears.

Your throat is dry and scratchy, mucous membranes are dry, your get frequent nosebleeds, especially in the winter. You also seem to catch any cold or aliment that passes by.

Eyes appear sunken, you don't sweat, and urine is scant and dark in color.

When pinched in a fold, the skin holds the shape, isn't elastic and doesn't bounce back. Blood pressure readings are low.

The entire system is working overtime just to try to maintain equilibrium without water. Skin feels dry, tight, flakes and breaks out in rashes easily when mild dehydration is long term.

Because water helps regulate the body temperature, in some cases of dehydration, there is fever. In all cases of fever, keep an eye on fluid intake because fever uses up water in the body at a high rate as it attempts to cool down.

The body releases water through the skin to cool the system. The evaporation of the water, as it is exposed to air, provides cooling. When there is no water to release, the body does not get the cooling action it needs and the body's core temperature can rise.

Serious cases of untreated dehydration can lead to delirium, unconsciousness and even death. It's nothing to take lightly.

You should never give fluids to anyone who has passed out, for any reason. It's time to call 911 and let the professionals take over.

The best news is that even moderate dehydration can easily be treated by drinking more water or electrolyte rich fluids. There are some simple recipes later in this book for an electrolyte drink and other refreshing beverages in addition to high hydrating foods that provide decent levels of fluid to the system.

We already mentioned muscles are 75% water. When muscles are dehydrated, they become cramped, tired, weak, and fatigued. The brain being between 85% and 90% water shows symptoms through mild headaches and difficulty focusing.

The blood being 83% water uses the fluid to move nutrients and waste products through and out of the body. When toxins are in the kidneys, proper hydration ensures fast processing and removal of toxins. If dehydrated, these same toxins become concentrated and remain in contact with the various organs involved in the removal process longer because there is not enough fluid to move things along quickly. You can see how this lingered exposure can cause undesired problems like tumors, cancerous growth, infections and other problems.

In Dr. Natasha Campbell-McBride's book, *GAPS Gut and Psychology Syndrome,* she discusses the effects of gut disease on the entire body. In her book, she discusses the development of tumors due to the overexposure to toxins and slow elimination, mostly partial and not complete, which results in further complicating issues. These issues lead to medical procedures and other developments that include odd poking, prodding and sticking, and inserting things with invasive procedures; all this is totally unnecessary if good health and hydration is maintained.

Emerging research is showing a connection between the health of the gut and the health of the body. While we have been taught the brain is the most important organ, research is demonstrating areas where the brain takes commands from the gut, rather than the other way around. It is emerging, cutting edge research that commands attention.

Bones are 22% water; the cartilage protecting the joints is over 80% water. Cartilage is slicker than ice which provides the perfect surface for bones to glide without damage. When dehydrated, the surface of the cartilage can get scratched, torn or damaged as it becomes brittle from lack of hydration. This commonly leads to joint replacement and injections or other procedures to lessen the constant pain of bone on bone contact.

To function at its best, the stomach lining needs to be fully hydrated at 98% water. The stomach lining provides a thick mucus cushion that is alkaline in nature that resists the acid production of the stomach through the bicarbonate it produces. If this lining becomes thin, weak or develops holes, acid reflux, peptic ulcers and other stomach ailments prevail. Instead of reaching for an antacid, try a glass of water.

Pay attention to when you drink too. You don't want to dilute the stomach acid too much during the digestion process. Drink only enough to comfortably swallow food during a meal. Consume larger amounts of fluids between meals.

Mild dehydration can cause you to lose focus and have difficulty making good decisions. It can be the cause for your afternoon slump and that nagging headache or muscle cramps.

A study at the busy University of Washington showed that a glass of water can shut down hunger pangs in most dieters. If you diet, isn't this worth a try?

5. HOW MUCH SHOULD YOU DRINK?

When asked, most people respond with "Well, I've been told eight to ten glasses per day." Then further examination reveals they think that means eight to ten glasses of whatever glass is sitting in front of them, which is typically a rather large glass or drinking device.

When faced with the prospect of drinking eight to ten glasses of twenty or thirty-two ounces per glass or cup, that is rather daunting.

Naturally, all kinds of excuses pop up.

Do you recognize any of these?

- "I can't drink that much
- I don't like the taste of water
- I'd be peeing all day!
- Water makes me feel full so I can't eat my meals
- Water is hard to swallow
- I'll get bloated
- I heard it's bad to drink that much!
- I'm NOT giving up my favorite soda!! (Or sweet tea, "energy drink" etc.)

- Give my water to thirsty children in Africa, I'm not drinking it.

And the excuses go on and on. But honestly, I think the health industry can do much more to create an understanding of how much water we really do need to drink on a daily basis. There should be at least, a clear, easy to understand idea, which is the mission of this book.

There are no "Official Guidelines" but there is plenty of advice out there. Just like children don't come with instruction booklets, neither do we get an instruction manual on how to take care of our inner workings. We just figure it out as we go along, depending on what we hear the most being the accepted fact and normal.

Most people do no research whatsoever when it comes to how to nourish and care for the body. We believe what we hear through clever marketing ploys from big food companies.

Remember the Wonder Bread Slogan?

"Helps Build Strong Bodies 12 Ways!"

Everyone actually believed this product, Wonder Bread, was good for their health and development when it had the nutritional value of tissue paper.

You know by now that the body is about 65-75% water. You know how the body uses water and the pros and cons of hydration vs. dehydration.

Now it is time get down to how you can take control and realistically consume the precious liquid your body needs to function at its best.

For instance a 120 pound person would need to drink 60 ounces a day for proper hydration.

THE FORMULA IS SIMPLE:

> *1/2 ounce for every pound you weigh or half your body weight in ounces.*

That seems like a lot. Break it down throughout the day. How many hours are you awake during an average day? Between twelve to fourteen hours is typical. If you divide those 60 ounces by 12 or 14, you will discover that between four to five ounces per hour will easily satisfy this quota.

That works out to be ½ of a cup or ½ cup plus a generous mouthful each hour you are awake. Most drinking cups and glasses are between eight and twenty-four ounces. A glass used for "on the rocks" style drinks is about eight ounces for a quick measure.

> 2 Tablespoons of water will equal 1 ounce
> 2 ounces of water will equal ¼ cup
> 4 ounces of water will equal ½ cup
> 8 ounces of water will equal 1 cup

Every cell in the body uses water; it is the primary building block of cells. Every system in the body depends upon water to function properly. Miraculously, the body will take water from itself to ensure survival, sacrificing the least important as it chooses what to protect.

This book is the closest thing you are going to find to a simple maintenance manual for your body. The rules are quite simple: drink and eat your water each and every day, move so you can, and be grateful and keep moving.

If you only do one thing, drinking water, you will notice a big improvement in your basic health. However, if you are under a doctor's care or on medication, please consult with your medical care team before you just go off and start drinking more water than you ever have.

Did You Know...?

It is possible to over hydrate just as it is to under hydrate.

6. OVER-HYDRATION

Yes, it is possible to overhydrate by drinking too much water. Water intoxication and another condition caused by water intoxication, hyponatremia, are serious issues and can lead to death.

The blood is a delicate balance of electrolytes which is a balance of seven major elements:

- Sodium (Na+)
- Chloride (Cl-)
- Potassium (K+)
- Magnesium (Mg++)
- Calcium (Ca++)
- Phosphate (HPO4—)
- Bicarbonate (HCO3-)

Each has a positive or negative charged atom that separates in water to create a charged environment. The balance between electrolytes is delicate.

Too much sodium in the diet can lead to high blood pressure and other organ damage. Too little sodium and you experience hyponatremia, a problem from too much water and not enough sodium.

Electrolyte imbalance can cause irregular heartbeat, tissue swelling leading to cell rupture, fluid in the lungs, fluttering eye lids. The behavior is much like that of someone being drunk or even drowning due to the swelling pressure on the brain and nerves. If the brain continues to swell, seizures, coma and death may occur unless water intake is restricted or a heavy saline solution is administered.

Full recovery in a few days can be expected unless the tissue swelling caused too much cellular damage.

> *In the kitchen we can see cellular damage caused by over marinating. If you leave a piece of steak in Worcestershire sauce or chicken or pork in citrus juices, you can see and feel the breakdown of the meat. On a molecular level what has happened is the cells absorbed as much as they could, then ruptured. This is bad news. It leaves the meat mushy and mealy, really unappetizing.*

If you drink more than six to eight ounces of water with your meals, you dilute the stomach acids to the point of not being able to digest the food properly. When the food is churned through the system, it may not be digested enough to extract sufficient nutrients and the system will have to work harder to continue the incomplete process. You will feel gas, bloating and diarrhea and experience nutrient deficiencies.

Remember not enough water reduces the stomach lining, which is rich in bicarbonate, which protects our stomach from the acid. At 98% water, it is essential to stay hydrated to keep the lining at peak performance.

Too much water dilutes the system; not enough depletes it; you've got to maintain the balance.

Are you at risk for water intoxication? Not really, mostly babies fed an over diluted formula or athletes who don't pace consumption during a big race or event are at the highest risk.

Parents should not over-dilute formula and athletes should sip small amounts of water, ice chips or electrolyte replenishing drinks that are sugar, chemical and dye free throughout the race instead of all at one time. It's the overload that causes problems.

For non-infant or extreme athlete persons, which means normal folks, if you are thirsty, drink a glass of water; wait five minutes and drink another. Chances are you'll stop feeling thirsty after the second glass. The average person would either vomit the excess water or expel it in urine rather quickly.

Athletes can keep water intoxication at bay by drinking fluids that replenish electrolytes instead of plain water and to sip steadily rather than gulp sporadically.

A normal healthy adult has kidneys that can process fifteen liters of water per day. However, the kidneys cannot process all of that liquid at one time. Choosing to distribute fluid consumption throughout the day is the best choice to make.

You must keep in mind too, that you can get up to 20% of your daily hydration needs from the foods you eat, which is what we look at in the next chapter. Hydration from food is the key the survival of some.

Did You Know...?

The kangaroo rat does not need to drink water. It gets 100% of its daily hydration needs from the food it eats on a daily basis.

7. HIGH HYDRATING FOODS

To those who do not like drinking water, it is almost a relief to hear that 20% of your daily water requirements can be satisfied by the foods you eat every day.

You may be surprised to see what the top hydrating foods are and why some are higher on the list than others.

This brief list illustrates how hydrating some foods actually are.

Do you realize that cauliflower provides more water than watermelon?

All of the foods we discuss in this chapter are 90% or more water. The best part is that they also are rich in vitamins, minerals, fiber and flavor.

At the end of the chapter is a chart of all the food discussed so you can be sure to choose these foods over others when you are planning meals.

If you care for someone who has a hard time swallowing liquids, you will want to choose foods for them from this list to help them get as much water into their systems as possible.

When you look at the list, it appears that you can make a really good salad for a meal or even part of one, to satisfy this 20% of water from the foods you eat. Take cucumber, it contains the most water of all. It's like crunchy water.

CUCUMBER   96.7%

Howard Murad MD, author of *The Water Secret* says that "eating three ounces of cucumber is like drinking three ounces of water, but better."

Why is it better? Instead of just getting water, you are also getting nutrients and fiber when you eat the cucumber. It provides potassium and a trace of magnesium which work with sodium to regulate body fluids and temperature. Remember those electrolytes? Cucumbers are also rich in Vitamin C, Vitamin K and some B vitamins as well as several other nutrients.

Interestingly enough, cucumbers contain the highest amount of water of any solid food and are one of the healthiest you can eat. Think about a cucumber being over 96% water while you eat it… this is why they do not freeze well. You could, but there wouldn't be much left once defrosted. This is also why when it is cut, cubed, sliced or blended, over time the water seeps out of the cut cell structure thusly creating a watery sauce, salsa or salad.

To use cucumbers in recipes like Tzatziki Sauce, cut cucumbers then drain them for at least an hour. After you drain them, fold the cucumber into the rest of your sauce and your sauce will not turn watery. Use the drained juice in water for a refreshing beverage or put it into a spritz bottle and use it as a cooling body spray.

Cucumbers have a great cellular structure that allows them to absorb vinegar and other flavors easily. This is why cucumbers make great pickles; a crunchy, seasoned, fermented vinegar delivery device.

Yum.

ICEBERG LETTUCE   95.6%

Butter-head, Green Leaf and Romaine are far better choices when basing your lettuce choice upon nutrients. But you cannot beat the water content of the much shunned Iceberg Lettuce. In cuisine, it does have its place as it provides a sharp bitter flavor that complements burgers and tuna salad so very well. It is also a great delivery device for blue cheese dressing and Asian Lettuce Wraps are simply divine when wrapped in Iceberg leaves.

Iceburg lettuce provides Vitamins B-6, thiamin and folate (both B vitamins) Vitamin C, and Vitamin K. Iceberg mainly provides over 95% water and dietary fiber. This is a great summer lettuce!

Don't think of Iceberg Lettuce as being low in nutrients but rather as being lower in nutrients than other choices.

If delivering water is your objective, this lettuce is your choice.

CELERY   95.4%

Celery provides potassium, Vitamin C and Vitamin A, is water rich, and provides a nice amount of fiber per stalk. All you have to do is eat a stalk that hasn't been de-strung to notice the fiber.

The drawback of celery is that each stalk also provides about 88 mgs of salt which is about 4% of your daily allowance. This makes celery naturally high in sodium, so you need to be aware of that. At only six calories per stalk, you can cut back on adding salt somewhere else.

Celery provides a great crunch and is a good replacement to help satisfy crunchy cravings. Dip into hummus or ginger miso dressing for some ideas. With the high fiber, adding protein like nut butters help satisfy hunger pangs and hold off the feeling of hunger longer than something with less fiber. Just be mindful of the salt and no canned spray cheese! Decide to choose low sodium dips and spreads.

Dried celery powder is used as a natural nitrite when curing meats without traditional curing salts. During the curing process the dried celery powder forms a natural nitrite that has the same preservation effect as the chemicals used in commercial curing of bacon, jerky, etc.

Why does celery make a good curing component? Because celery it is naturally high in sodium, remember?

RADISHES   95.3%

Radishes are a great little package of heat, and sometimes sweet, hit of crunch. They are a powerhouse of hydration and flavor. Radishes of all kinds should be in just about every summer salad.

I adore radishes for breakfast. When in France, we get a fresh baguette, some cheese, charcuterie or a roasted chicken, some fresh radishes, French butter, fleur de sel and a bottle of wine and go have a picnic in the park. The freshness of the radishes really sets the meal off. (Or could it have been that we were in France?)

Wash and have them handy for the crunchy craving; lightly sprinkle them with Himalayan Pink Salt which is also very rich with over eighty vitamins and minerals.

Slice any variety of radish thin and pop them onto a sandwich for some fun. One of my favorite sandwiches is ham, Dijon, butter, and radish with cornichons (French sour pickles) on the side.

Be adventurous and steam radishes; serve them with butter, salt and pepper, just as you would a turnip or rutabaga. You can call them baby pink turnips, just to be fancy.

Steamed and buttered red radishes are tremendous with lamb. Just be aware that at 95% water, they do not puree well. They turn into a watery mess instead.

All radishes are a good source of Riboflavin, Vitamin B6, Calcium, Magnesium, Copper and Manganese, and a very good source of Dietary Fiber, Vitamin C, Folate and Potassium.

TOMATOES   94.5%

All varieties of tomatoes are excellent sources of antioxidants, dietary fiber, minerals, and vitamins. All varieties from the grape, cherry, Roma type and the amazing Heirloom varieties available are all a great resource. Tomatoes are rich in variety, flavor and nutrients.

The antioxidants present in tomatoes are scientifically found to be protective against cancers, including colon, prostate, breast, endometrial, lung, and pancreatic tumors.

Lycopene, a flavonoid antioxidant, is a unique phytochemical compound found in the tomatoes. It is said to be good for the eyes and also for the skin.

Did you know…?

Red fruits tend to possess more of this antioxidant than other fruits. As with all fruits and vegetables, choose those with the darkest colors for the most concentration of nutrients.

Zea-xanthin is a flavonoid compound we seldom hear about that is abundant in tomatoes. Zea-xanthin helps protect eyes from age-related macular disease by filtering ultra-violet rays from the sun.

Tomatoes contain good levels of vitamin A, and flavonoid anti-oxidants xanthins and lutein. Altogether, these pigment compounds are found to have antioxidant properties and take part in night-vision, maintenance of healthy mucus membranes, skin, and bones.

Tomatoes are also good source of antioxidant Vitamin-C, rich in potassium and just 5 mg of sodium. Potassium is an important component of cell and body fluids that helps to control heart rate and blood pressure caused by sodium; electrolytes at work again.

Further, tomatoes carry normal levels of B-complex vitamins such as folates, thiamin, niacin, riboflavin as well some essential minerals like iron, calcium, manganese and other trace elements.

Whether you eat them cooked or raw, tomatoes are a sure bet for flavor and value in your diet.

Research regarding zea-xanthan is emerging and can easily be found and followed on the internet. There are several links in the Appendix to the research used to write this book.

BELL PEPPERS, GREEN   93.9%

All bell peppers are rich in vitamins A and C, potassium and fiber. Peppers can be sweet or they can pack a punch of heat as in jalapeno or ghost peppers. Green peppers are picked before they have a chance to turn yellow or red or orange therefore they have slightly higher water content.

BELL PEPPERS, RED OR YELLOW   92%

Sweet peppers that are red, yellow or orange have higher 1 ½ times more vitamin C and red peppers pack the highest amount of nutrition in them because they have been on the plant the longest. Green peppers are harvested earlier; the colored peppers are left on the plant longer.

Did you know?

Cutting fresh peppers is easy when you place the skin side down on the cutting board. The knife grips and glides through the flesh side of the pepper easier than the skin side. The skin side is slick and may cause the knife to slip and could cause an injury.

CAULIFLOWER   92.1%

Packed with Vitamin C and beta-carotene, this is one powerhouse of a vegetable. Being a cruciferous vegetable, it has so many health benefiting compounds, you would do well to eat cauliflower often.

It's also nice to see it is high in water. This is why, when trying to make Paleo pizza crusts or "breads" from cauliflower, you need to squeeze the water out of it after it has been cooked in order to actually make it into a substance that can be used for a pizza crust. Chopped cauliflower can be substituted for rice and it also makes an amazing smooth and delicious puree or soup.

Popular recipes use steamed or simmered cauliflower, pureed, as a delicious substitute for mashed potatoes. I think that if you are going to mash cauliflower and call it mashed potatoes, you should warn people or else they'll think you make the worst mashed potatoes in the world. Cauliflower and potatoes do not taste similar and I adore them both.

Try cooking cauliflower in chamomile tea for amazing flavor enrichment.

Keep an eye out for our Healthy & Hydrated Workshops where you can learn many different recipes using high hydration foods.

WATERMELON   91.5%

This refreshing summertime treat needs to have another thought. At nearly 92% water, this robust melon supplies us with significant levels of Vitamins A and C and amino acids like lycopene which is a huge antioxidant.

The darker pink-red the flesh is, the higher the lycopene content. Researchers found that light/white fleshed watermelons contain very low levels if any lycopene at all. Why is lycopene important? It helps you deal with stress. Watermelon is anti-inflammatory, it rehydrates and also provides fiber.

Recent research shows watermelon is also high in the amino acid citrulline, which the body converts to another amino acid, arginine. These amino acids and their conversions are very helpful with blood circulation and cardiovascular health.

The down side of watermelon, however, is the sugar content. It is naturally high in sugar so be aware.

Using watermelon in place of tomatoes to create Gazpacho is an attention grabbing recipe. Simply use watermelon anywhere the recipe calls for tomato.

Other savory favorites include a salad made from Feta cheese and onions or grilling watermelon.

Yes, I said grilled watermelon with olive oil, herbs de Provence and Maldon salt. (Screaming hot grill, slap the melon down, grill till it just marks the melon. Cross hatch if you like, I like stripes on my grilled watermelon.)

I dare you to try it!

SPINACH   91.4%

Your skin, hair and bones will thank you for eating spinach, raw or cooked. Spinach is high in vitamin K, & A, potassium and magnesium as well as many other powerful nutrients. It is considered a functional food because it is anti-inflammatory, and some say it can reduce the risk of cancer.

All greens, collards, Swiss chard, kale are like putting pure gold into your body when you eat them. Strive to eat greens, cooked or raw every day.

STAR FRUIT AKA CARAMBOLA   91.4%

These amusing fruits are quite tasty and are a great visual interest at well. When you cut these fruits the slices are star shaped. Do you remember the cartoon "Winky Dink?"

Carambola grows in subtropical climates. High in vitamin C and a host of other nutrients, this sweet/tart fruit will capture your taste buds.

As with all fruit, it is best eaten when ripe. To save yourself a puckered, severe fish face when you eat a slice, you need to make sure the fruit is ripe. When ripe, the fruit will be yellow and the five ribs will have brown edges, not green. Green means it isn't quite ready to eat yet.

If you do eat star fruit with green ribs, you'll wish you waited. Do you remember those horrible super sour candies, popular a while back? Sour, like that. It is worth the wait for the brown edges.

Trust me.

When I lived in South Florida, we had a friend who had two carambola trees in her yard. We had boxes of carambola and tried nearly everything there was to be made with them. My favorite is fresh, sliced; warm from the sun and fresh from the tree.

STRAWBERRIES   91%

Please, please buy organic strawberries! Commercially grown berries have so many chemicals and pesticides, and they have no flavor.

Here's the line-up: Vitamin C, folate, manganese and potassium and high in dietary fiber. These juicy, sweet fruits have great power to lower blood pressure and to lower your risk for certain cancers.

The Environmental Working Group (EWG) just released the latest list of produce that is the most contaminated with pesticides and for the first time in four years, commercially grown strawberries top the list with up to thirteen different chemicals and pesticides found on and in the berries.

What did strawberries knock down the list?

Apples.

What can you do?

Buy organic. Demand organic; because it does matter.

I was at a food event recently, several vendors displaying their wares and promoting their products. One table was about fresh produce. When I asked about their organic availability, the young girl working the table told me that the organic option was possible.

She had strawberries to taste and when I asked her if they were organic, she responded that she didn't understand why people make such a fuss over organic. Strawberries are strawberries except when a commercially grown strawberry gets over three hundred pounds of chemicals per acre that leaves residue of over thirteen pesticides, weed killers and other chemicals on and in the berries, I do think it matters.

I do not believe there is EVER a time when it is good to eat those kinds of food.

And I wonder if store workers sell or mark items as organic when they are not. Stickers and tape come off things.

See the appendix of this book for a complete list of the *EWG Dirty Dozen and Clean Fifteen.*

BROCCOLI   90.7%

Another highly beneficial vegetable, broccoli has the highest protein content of vegetables. Being a member of the cruciferous family, along with cabbage, kale and cauliflower, this is another extremely power packed vegetable.

While broccoli can be eaten raw, it supplies the best and most nutrients when it has been lightly steamed. Broccoli provides Vitamins C, K folate, dietary fiber and iron and potassium. Regular consumption of broccoli has proven to benefit blood circulation, heart health and the health of the eyes.

At 90% water, the protein found in broccoli is considered low, but it's high when looking at protein in vegetables. 1 cup provides 3 grams of protein.

Buy organic whenever possible. I can taste the difference between conventional broccoli and organic.

Organic broccoli tastes like broccoli should: full, rich and flavorful.

GRAPEFRUIT   90.5%

Ever since I was young people have talked about "The Grapefruit Diet." As a hybrid member of the citrus family, grapefruit has long been touted for its ability to help drop the pounds by simply drinking a glass of grapefruit juice every day. Doing so, several of those unwanted pounds would simply melt away. Of course it didn't happen that way and many women got mouth ulcers and irritated stomachs from drinking too much grapefruit juice.

Grapefruit is a tricky one in that it can react with so many medications. Before you go off and start drinking grapefruit juice or scarfing down entire grapefruits for breakfast, check with your doctor to see if there are any side affects you should know about.

Once you get the clear for consuming grapefruit, enjoy many colors. The darker red versions provide more lycopene and vitamin C. The lighter colored fruits have lesser amounts of lycopene.

As with all citrus, consume in moderation. Over consumption of citrus fruits, including lemon juice, lime juice; have been known to cause mouth sensitivity, small blisters or ulcers and erosion of tooth enamel.

The citric acid can be strong and have effects so moderation is the key.

BABY CARROTS   90.4%

Baby carrots have more water than regular carrots. Why?

Because baby carrots are scraped into shape (shock, I know) and in order to keep them shapely and lovely orange and other colors for your viewing and eating pleasure, they need to be in a bit of water.

If the scraped carrots were not in water, they would dry out and develop white patches on the outside of the carrot where the skin was scraped away. You'd never buy them.

Marketers are clever.

So the baby carrots are scraped into shapes and packaged in a bit of water to keep them "fresh" looking. Because of this, they also absorb some of that water thereby making them higher in water content than regular carrots. This makes them attractive so you'll buy them and cute so you'll eat them.

Serve carrots raw for a great snappy snack.

Rich in beta carotene, carrots are good for your eyes, skin and liver.

CANTALOUPE   90.2%

High in antioxidants Vitamins A and C, in addition to vitamin K, potassium, magnesium and dietary fiber, this melon is a perennial hit.

A bowl of cantaloupe is only about 50 calories and at 90% water is sure to satisfy both a sweet tooth and part of your hydration needs. Here's a Big Bonus: a single six-ounce serving of cantaloupe provides

100% of your daily Vitamin C and A requirement.

Did you know…?

A cantaloupe will taste like it smells? Sniff the end where it was attached to the vine. Buy what smells good.

Melons should be heavy for their size.

So there you have it; some of the highest water content foods you can buy on a regular basis. All should be readily available with the exception of the Star Fruit. If star fruit (carambola) isn't common to your area, keep an eye out for it when you travel or have some sent to you. When fully ripe, they are a real treat.

CHART OF HIGH HYDRATING FOODS

Cucumber	96.7%
Iceberg Lettuce	95.6%
Celery	95.4%
Radishes	95.3%
Tomatoes	94.5%
Green Peppers	93.9%
Red or yellow peppers	92%
Cauliflower	92.1%
Watermelon	91.5%
Spinach	91.4%
Star Fruit	91.4%
Strawberries	91%
Broccoli	90.7%
Grapefruit	90.5%
Baby Carrots	90.4%
Cantaloupe	90.2%

8. IN CASE YOU WANT TO KNOW: ELECTROLYTES & ANTIOXIDANTS

Electrolytes and antioxidants are things you hear thrown around all the time now when talking about health, diet and nutrition. Do you ever wonder electrolytes or antioxidants are or what a free radical is?

The body is amazing. If you are curious, read on. If not, skip to the next chapter after you drink ½ cup of water.

What are electrolytes and antioxidants anyway? In layman's terms, how do they work?

A brief explanation of electrolytes:

Our bodies have seven components that are electronically charged and provide the important function of balancing blood pressure, muscle contraction and heartbeat, which is essentially muscle contraction.

The Seven Electrolyte Components:

1. **Sodium** – found on the outside of out cells. Sodium is one half of the electrolyte pump that keeps the system in balance,

regulating blood pressure, muscle contractions and heartbeat.

2. **Chloride** – works closely with sodium to balance extracellular fluids.

3. **Potassium** – found on the inside of our cells. Potassium is vitally important as the other half of the electrolyte pump. Potassium controls heartbeat, muscle function such as in the lungs. As well as Potassium also ensures the ability of the cells to communicate with each other. Too much potassium in the body can be fatal and must be dealt with quickly by medical professionals. Too little potassium is easily solved: eat a banana.

4. **Magnesium** – the most underappreciated electrolyte. Magnesium plays an important role in the synthesis of DNA and RNA of every living thing on the planet. It also regulates heartbeat, blood pressure and the nervous system.

5. **Calcium** – is found in the bones, teeth and nails but also in trace quantities in our nerves and blood plasma. It is essential to blood clotting.

6. **Phosphate** – After calcium, phosphate is the most abundant mineral in your body. It plays an important role in cellular repair and works closely with calcium to strengthen bones, nails and teeth.

7. **Bicarbonate** – works to provide a buffering system, helping to keep the ph. levels of our blood steady and where they should be. The kidneys control the release of bicarbonate to steady the alkaline or acid conditions of the system.

A brief explanation of antioxidants:

Antioxidants are the vitamins A, C, E, beta carotene and lycopene.

It sounds almost like learning grade school grammar. While antioxidants aren't actually *things* like vitamins A, C, and E, antioxidants *influence a particular kind of behavior* between cells that make them antioxidants. So rather than being a thing, antioxidants are more about how cells behave and treat each other.

Cells can become damaged through oxidizing leaving them with broken or missing atoms that make them unpredictable, and simply put, behave badly. These cells become bullies. They try to steal the atoms they need from perfectly good neighbors in an attempt to stabilize their own instability.

These bad cells are called free radicals and they have a bad influence on other good cells, causing perfectly good cells to turn around and behave badly as well. This can cause a downward spiral that leads to disease, cancers and all kinds of other negative things that can happen to the body.

The cells try to stabilize themselves before they reproduce because if they reproduce with broken or missing bits of atoms, they reproduce exactly like the damaged cell, not a healthy one. This is not a good thing; you need healthy cells, not damaged ones.

This is where the antioxidants come into play. Antioxidants lend free radicals the atoms they are missing or have damaged thereby making the free radical cells behave better by not stealing from their neighbors which would have started a chain reaction of bad behavior. By not stealing, the nearby cells are safe from damage caused by free radicals.

Plain and simple, antioxidants help damaged cells by giving them what they need in order not to damage other good cells surrounding it.

Research has also proven that taking an abundance of antioxidants shows no singular beneficial effect against aging. Antioxidants are part of a very complex program and work best in conjunction with total nutrition and show no improved performance by overloading these nutrients.

I would like to make animated movies to illustrate these points because I believe that if we understood how our bodies function, we would treat them better. We need to do better educating people about health.

I once had a young client who was pregnant. I asked her to keep a food journal because she said she was having issues keeping her energy up.

When she shared her journal with me I noticed that on several days the only thing she ate all afternoon was an entire bag of Sour Cream and Onion potato chips. When we talked about it she told me she thought it was the same as eating a baked potato without having to "cook it the normal way."

Needless to say, we had some serious lessons on good food. She appreciated it and declared that she simply did not know because no one had ever taught her anything about food.

Start somewhere and learn all you can about the food you put into your body.

9. HOW AND WHEN TO DRINK WATER

Believe it or not, there is a way to drink water for maximum benefit. There are times you should imbibe generously and other times when you should sip just enough to keep things lubricated.

Let me explain.

Your body uses water constantly. You lose up to eight ounces of water overnight just through breathing and body temperature regulation. If you were to drink your entire daily water requirement at one time, your body would use what it needs *at that time* and then get rid of the rest through urine or vomit.

If you were to drink too much at one time, there is danger of water intoxication. The acid and electrolyte balance would become totally off kilter and this can lead to death, so it is not a good idea. The opposite of water intoxication is dehydration and by now, we should know something about dehydration too. (Refer to chapters four and six)

So what is the best way to consume the water we need on a daily basis? Here is an easy list to get you started. If you do not implement everything, decide to start somewhere and improve as you get used to your hydration program.

Here are a few suggestions:

1. Make it a habit. Calculate what your daily need is and then measure it out. Find a water bottle you can carry with you; mark it off so you have a visual of how much water you have drunk and still need to drink each day.

    When I refer to a glass of water, I use the standard measure of eight ounces or one cup. You can choose the standard measure that suits you. Some use ten ounces because it is easily divisible. I prefer using the eight ounce measure because it is an easy couple of swallows.

2. Drink your first glass while you are waiting for the coffee to brew or as soon as you get up in the morning.

3. Drink water every couple of hours but stop drinking thirty minutes before a meal. To lose weight, drink an eight ounce glass of water thirty minutes before a meal, then wait for the meal. The stomach will recognize that you are eating about twenty minutes after you start eating. If you have a glass of water thirty minutes before you start eating, your stomach thinks it is already eating by the time you actually do start filling up.

4. Start your meal with a light soup or salad. Then by the time you get to your more dense foods like meat, pasta, bread etc., your stomach is already registering full so you will consume fewer of these foods.

5. With a meal only drink six to eight ounces during the meal, just enough to wash things down. Drinking too much at mealtime dilutes the stomach acid and makes it very hard to digest food

properly.

6. To lose weight, drink eight ounces of water thirty minutes before a meal. This will trigger your brain into thinking your stomach is filling up before you begin eating. Remember your brain will recognize that you are eating about twenty minutes after you start filling your stomach. Pace your food during the first twenty minutes so you do not over eat. See tip number four.

7. To keep from having to wake up during the night to use the bathroom, make it a goal to have consumed all of your DWR by dinner time.

Once you get in the habit of drinking what you need, it becomes second nature.

Let me remind you of all the health benefits you will gain from consuming your daily water requirement.

- You can lose weight; drinking water reduces hunger
- That nagging headache will go away
- Your skin will look younger
- Your skin will have a youthful glow
- Your body will perform better while exercising
- Your digestion system will function better
- Fewer sprains and cramps in your muscles
- You will be healthier
- You will have more energy
- Your mood will be great
- Your cancer risk is lessened
- Sex will be better; your skin will feel wonderful to your partner.

- People will wonder what you are up to
- Your confidence will soar!
- You will get more done because you will have more energy
- Your mind will be sharper; you will think clearer and be able to focus better.
- You will be able to develop more projects and new ideas with ease because of your mental clarity
- You will feel great in your skin, inside and out

Makes you thirsty, right?

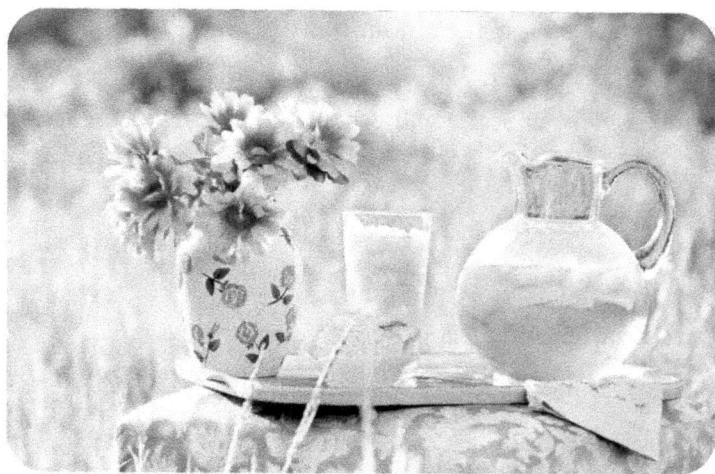

10.   REFRESHING BEVERAGES

Here you will find some basic suggestions for creating a refreshing beverage that everyone will crave and really look forward to drinking.

The secret is to back off the amount of sugar used so your beverage is not a sugar laden disaster. Most of the time the beverages will taste great all on their own but some will prefer a touch of sweetener, which is fine, as long as it is not a lot of sugar and the sugar used is natural and not artificial.

Artificial sweeteners should be avoided at all costs.

Imagine your body as a machine again, with your skin performing its job of cooling the body by sweating. Think of how different that machine would function if it were fueled with pure clean liquids or those laden with sugar and cream, artificial colors, dyes and fake flavors? In the former scenario the skin is left with a trace of salt but clean feeling while if your body has to deal with sugar drinks, it is just not as good, not as easy, to process.

Here are a few recipes to play with just to get you started making your own refreshing beverages. Change the fruit, change the tea, and change the herbs or flowers; the combinations are limitless. Mix it up a bit and do not be afraid to play with combinations.

A Note about Using Citrus

When steeping citrus peel, only steep a short time to avoid the bitter flavor development from the white pith found under the colored peel. Alternatively, zest citrus before steeping, using only the colored part of the citrus skin; discarding the white pith.

If garnishing with slices of lemon, lime, grapefruit or orange, always remove the fruit slices before storing overnight. If you do not, the beverage will become quite bitter.

There is a popular practice to drink lemon juice in water every morning as you start the day. While there are many health benefits to this practice, it would be a good idea to consult your dentist for the best advice regarding your teeth.

Lemon water can cause erosion of the tooth enamel over time. Your best choice is to find a beverage you can alternate, a pinch of Himalayan salt in water would be a viable alternative to everyday lemon water. It is the acid that is the concern.

Consult your dentist for advice on your teeth and oral health as it relates to the drinking of lemon juice.

Disposal of Steeped Material

Because I like to connect with the earth, I compost the ingredients used for refreshing beverages. I honor the service to my body and health then put the debris back into the cycle of life.

Teas

Making tea is more of a process than an actual thing. Tea can be made from anything that can be soaked in hot water for a while to extract flavor. It is not necessarily a call to grab the orange pekoe teabags. You can make tennis shoe tea although it would not be very pleasant.

To make tea from citrus peel, pour boiling water directly over the peels or zest. Allow to steep 5 minutes then strain. Reserve the liquid for your refreshing beverages.

To make tea from other things: Simply use about a handful of fresh herbs or fruit per quart of tea desired. Use actively boiling water to pour over the items and steep to desired strength. If you are not sure, taste it.

Simple Syrup

Making your own simple syrup ensures you know the quality of the sugar you are using and you can control how much is used.

Add high quality organic granulated sugar to a heavy bottomed pot. Add enough fresh, clean water to cover the sugar by about an inch. Eyeball this measure, no need to grab a ruler.

Did You Know...?

Your index and middle fingers together are approximately one inch, that's close enough for most measures. Unless you are cutting wood, of course.

Over high heat, stir the sugar and water to make sure it is all combined, bring to a boil then simmer for 3 minutes. Remove from heat, cool. Store Simple Syrup in the refrigerator until needed.

To make flavored Simple Syrup, add desired flavorings to the syrup while it is simmering. Strain to remove bits and pieces before using.

Examples of flavored Simple Syrup:

- Rosemary
- Basil
- Citrus zest (no pith): lemon, lime, orange, grapefruit, pomelo, kumquat
- Ginger
- Any fruit you like
- Any herb you like
- Sweet spices like cinnamon, cardamom
- Tomato (just try it)

The key is to experiment!

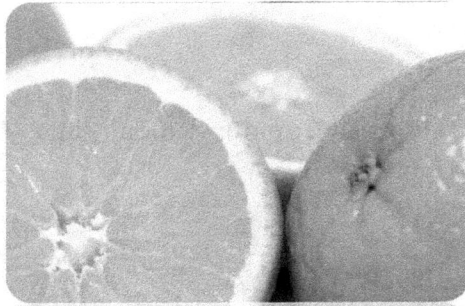

THE RECIPES:

Basic Lemonade:

- Fresh lemon juice
- Good Simple Syrup
- Clean water
- Lemon slices for garnish

Combine equal parts lemon juice and simple syrup; add enough water to dilute this by 75% or to your desired taste.

Example:

- *¼ cup lemon juice*
- *¼ cup simple syrup*
- *1-½ cups water*

Instead of drinking pure lemonade, use this to flavor other teas you drink to create quite unique beverages.

Lavender Lemonade

Pour 32 ounces of boiling water over 2 Tablespoons lavender buds. Steep for 5 minutes the strain and compost the lavender.

Put the lavender tea into a pitcher, to 32 ounces of lavender tea, add 8 ounces of fresh lemonade. Adjust flavor with clean cold water or sparkling water if you want bubbles.

Adjust the lemonade to taste, using it as the sweetener.

Example: To a tall iced tea glass add 1 cup lavender tea to ¼ cup lemonade. Fill with water and ice; adjust sweetener to desired taste.

This lemonade will help calm people down and make them feel good with less stress. It is unusual and delicious. Serve this at office meetings or when people are giving presentations or recitals. It has a great calming effect.

Hibiscus Lemonade

Pour 32 ounces of boiling water over ½ cup of dried hibiscus blossoms to make hibiscus tea. Let these steep as long as possible because they don't get bitter as they sit. You are going to adore the deep red color of this tea!

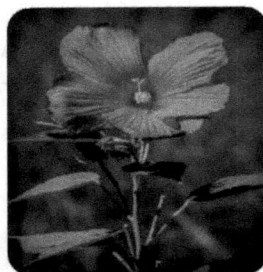

Pour the hibiscus tea into a pitcher or tall glass, add lemonade to taste. This is one you will eventually drink without any sweetener added. Hibiscus provides a high level of vitamin C and anthocyanins which are reported to help fight the development of cancer cells. By itself it has a tangy flavor almost similar to faint lemon.

Add lemonade to taste or sweeten as desired.

Serve hibiscus Tea hot or cold. Remember *Celestial Seasonings Red Zinger Tea?*

That is hibiscus.

Homemade Sports Drink: Electrolyte Fluid

This Electrolyte Beverage is for when you need more than just water. Make and drink this beverage when you have someone who is sick with fever, diarrhea, vomiting or someone who is doing exercise in the heat or even prolonged sports where muscles need more than plain water.

The Importance of Electrolytes

Water provides the medium for electrolytes to circulate throughout your body. Electrolytes are the minerals sodium, potassium, chloride, calcium and magnesium plus a few more. These electrolytes provide transportation of glucose and amino acids in and out of cells. Each electrolyte is balanced by another of equal but opposite charge to manage the flow of nutrients to cells and waste from cells and to help prevent muscle cramping. (See Chapter 8)

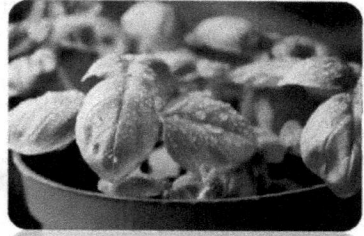

Ingredients

o 1/2 cup fresh orange juice

o 1/4 cup fresh lemon juice

o 2 cups of filtered water *or* raw coconut water

o 2 tablespoons organic raw honey or organic maple syrup

o 1/8 teaspoon Himalayan Pink salt (for its 85+ minerals)

Combine all ingredients and drink when the need to hydrate occurs. This drink is designed to replace Gatorade, PowerAde and all those chemical filled so-called hydrating beverages.

Make your own, know what is in it and feel the difference. I will bet you will not be missing those esters of wood rosin and artificial colors and flavors from your sports drink.

If you are doing an extreme sport where hydration is key; make this with coconut water rather than plain water. It will take you a whole lot further and your body will function really well.

Grapefruit Basil

Remove the zest from 1 grapefruit; place it into a teapot or large bowl. Add a generous handful of basil, stems and all; do not use the basil flowers because they are bitter. Pour 1 quart of boiling water over this and allow to steep for 5 minutes. Strain. Add the juice from the grapefruit and sweeten to taste. Pour over ice and garnish with a fresh basil leaf and a slice of grapefruit.

Ginger Lemon

Slice a lemon and place it into a bowl or teapot. Slice a 1 inch knob of fresh ginger or use 1 tablespoon for dried ginger, place this in the pot or bowl as well. Pour 1 quart of boiling water over this mixture and allow to steep 5-10 minutes.

Sweeten to taste if needed. Strain before serving hot or cold.

Garnish with a slice of lemon.

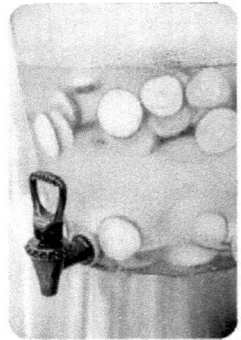

Strawberry Basil

Remove the tops from 1 cup of fresh strawberries, coarsely chop and place chopped berries into a bowl or teapot. Add a small handful of fresh basil with stems.

Pour 1 quart of boiling water over and allow to steep for 5-10 minutes.

Strain to remove seeds and debris; adjust sweetener if necessary.

Cucumber Water

Puree one cucumber; strain the liquids from the solids. Use the solids to make tzatziki sauce for a meal and use the water for a refreshing beverage.

Mix the cucumber juice with water, adjusting the dilution strength to taste. This beverage is not sweetened. Garnish with a thin slice or ribbon of cucumber.

Did You Know…?

To make a ribbon of cucumber: use a peeler to cut a long, thin slice from the length of the cucumber to use as a garnish.

Cucumber water makes a refreshing summer body spray, especially when it is chilled!

Mint tea

Take a generous amount of fresh mint, place it in a pot and cover it with boiling water. Allow to steep until it is cool. Strain and enjoy is a tall glass with ice. Sweeten to taste.

Plain mint tea makes an amazing hair rinse in the summer and also feels good in a spritz bottle on hot summer days. Just keep it out of your eyes; that would not be a good thing. Use unsweetened tea only as a body spray.

Chamomile Tea

Use fresh chamomile flowers or teabags, pour boiling water over and steep until cool. Drink plain or combine chamomile tea with hibiscus tea, sweeten to taste for an amazing beverage.

Chamomile has been used for centuries to help ease anxiety and to calm you down. It is especially useful to promote restful sleep.

Chamomile tea can be used to cook cauliflower, and then pureed to make a tasty soup. Remember that cauliflower is a high hydration food.

Attend a *Healthy & Hydrated Workshop* to learn how to make, taste and see to how Chamomile Cauliflower affects people in action. You want relaxed, happy people? Serve this soup with lavender lemonade.

Euphoria.

If your hair is blonde, or gray, use chamomile tea as a hair rinse to bring sparkle and shine to your hair.

Making Popsicles

All of these refreshing beverages can be made into delicious high hydrating popsicles. This can come in handy with children or someone who may have difficulty drinking fluids or is ill or bedridden.

Make the chosen beverage just a bit stronger than you normally would. Cool the liquid completely.

Taste your mixture to see if you like the flavor and adjust it while it cools.

Did You Know…?

Cold and frozen foods need to have stronger flavors than foods served hot. The cold masks the taste buds perception of flavor therefore cold foods need an added punch. Not just salt, but all flavors in the dish.

To make vegan popsicles, use coconut milk, almond milk or cashew milk or cream. I prefer to use plain Greek yogurt.

Plain Greek yogurt is thick and full of probiotics. Plain yogurt can be flavored according to choice with a variety of things from honey, agave, simple syrups, or fruit puree. Adding your own flavor gives you control over the amount of added sugar.

Combine the yogurt or other milk with the chosen beverage. Be sure to taste it! Pour into Popsicle molds and freeze.

The popsicles made with nut milks will be icier than those popsicles made with yogurt.

You can add thinly sliced fruit to the molds for flavor and variety. Think of a slice of kiwi with strawberry basil or chamomile with raspberries.

Pureed banana can also be used in place of yogurt or nut milk.

Popsicles are enjoyable and can be used to ease sore throats and provide hydration when ill. Popsicles are a great way to get some hydration into a busy, active child.

Of course you can just enjoy eating an amazing Popsicle too.

Let your imagination run wild!

11. CALCULATING YOUR DWR (DAILY WATER REQUIREMENT)

In this chapter you will find some worksheets to help you calculate and schedule your Daily Water Requirement (DWR) and intake.

Start a journal or keep record of how you feel as you increase your hydration. This one simple step can help prevent the onset of so many ailments and diseases.

Choose Health and Hydration!

Daily Water Requirement (DWR) Worksheet

Use this worksheet to calculate how much water you need each day.

Step 1: Accurately weigh yourself in pounds; without clothes, shoes, jewelry, etc.

My Weight:_____

Step 2: Divide your weight by 2

My Weight Divided by 2:_____

Step 3: Change the number in step 2 into ounces.

How much water I need to drink daily: _____ounces

Step 4: Subtract 20% from your DWR

(Select high hydration foods for up to 20% of your DWR)

MY TOTAL DWR: _____**Ounces**

Example:

Step 1: 120 pound person

Step 2: 120/2 = 60 pounds

Step 3: 60 pounds = 60 ounces

Step 4: 60 − 20% = 48 (60*.20=12; 60-12=48) Your DWR is 48 ounces

My DWR Consumption Schedule

Use this worksheet to schedule your water consumption. Once it becomes habit this schedule will create itself. Follow this worksheet to get you started.

Step 1: Determine your DWR minus the 20% allotment for hydrating foods.

Step 2: Divide your DWR by 10.

Step 3: Schedule drinking the amount determined in step 2 each hour for the next 10 hours.

Schedule appropriately around meal times and complete your consumption before evening hours so your sleep pattern is not interrupted by the need to use the bathroom.

Example:

DWR for 120 pound person is 60 ounces minus 20% for hydrating foods: 48 ounces

48/ 10 = 4.8 ounces each hour for 10 hours of being awake.

That is just a gulp over ½ cup of water each hour, which is totally doable. Of course you can drink more than that, but not too much more. If you are active you will need to consume more than someone with a sedentary lifestyle due to water loss from physical activity. Additionally, you will need to consume more if you live in a dry or hot environment.

Set a reminder until drinking water becomes a natural habit. Keep track of how much you drink all day so you learn to gage your consumption. Also, make note of how you feel physically and mentally.

You are going to love the way you feel.

Tip:

Start your day with an 8 ounce glass of room temperature water. Before coffee or tea; it's one of the best things you can do for your body in the morning.

Did you know that you take in more fluid when drinking from a straw?

The soft drink marketing industry certainly knows that

12. THE ENVIRONMENTAL IMPACT OF BOTTLED WATER

Now that you have come this far, you may be thinking about drinking some water. Please do not grab a plastic water bottle and make guzzling them your new habit.

Surely the marketing claims are "thinner plastic, less waste; recycled" but really, how many bottles of the billions produced are tossed away and not recycled and end up in landfills and trash piles. Fewer than 20% actually get recycled and those tops to the bottles? Not recyclable! This is one of the out of control effects of the frenzied bottled water consumption craze.

Did you know…?

It takes three times the amount of water to make a single plastic water bottle than it does to fill it?

We have been brainwashed by marketing to think of buying water in a bottle so you don't have to carry it around all day. Just drink, toss and go. We've been told bottled water is better for you. Truth is the bottle water industry is loosely regulated and the water coming from your taps, public water, is highly regulated, inspected and must meet particular standards. In fact, 40 percent of bottled water is simply bottled tap water that you have paid for through taxes. Manufacturers are bottling and selling it back to you at hugely inflated prices.

> *"It struck me that all you need to do is take water out of the ground and sell it for more than the price of wine, or for that matter, oil."*
>
> *Gustave Levin,*
> *Former Chairman of Perrier*

What happened in Flint, MI and other water municipalities is the people in control of the regulation were not doing their jobs. Now, they are being held accountable. The common citizen should be aware of the water situation in their area and speak up if you don't find something to your liking. Keep talking and engaging conversations until things change. That is what we do as Americans. We can change things.

To find out about the state of your public water supply where you live, contact your local water company. Ask for the *Annual Water Quality Report* which may be titled the *Consumer Confidence Report*. While these reports may be detailed and technical, they contain a lot of useful information about the water in your area.

While tap water isn't perfect, it is a regulated industry. The National Resources Defense Council surveyed random samples of bottled water only to confirm that 22% of the samples contained contaminate levels that exceeded state health mandates.

In taste tests conducted to see if people could tell the difference between bottled water and tap water, in the majority of cases, people could not tell the difference and often chose the tap water sample as the bottled water.

There are many options for putting a filtration system on the water you drink and use in your home. Personally, I prefer the reverse osmosis systems. They are easy to use, and provide a peace of mind for knowing the water you are drinking is as clean as possible.

Since nearly half of the bottled water on the shelves today is from the tap already, it makes sense to save money and resources by using a stainless steel or glass bottle or other reusable material for your water bottle. Refilling it is free and there is no waste! Win for you-win for the environment and win for the planet.

Here's the lowdown on plastic water bottles.

The older the plastic bottles become, the more chemicals leach into the water they contain. If the bottles are left in the sun or in a hot place where the temperatures get warm, as in your car or delivery truck, more chemicals are leached into the water inside the bottles.

This year alone, it will take seventeen billion barrels of oil to produce all the water bottles currently in demand. The bottled water industry has become a monster and an environmental disaster. Between bottled water and Keurig cups, there is a mad mission to destroy our planet in record time.

The Pacific Institute claims the cost would be the same to produce a bottle that contains one fourth pure oil as it is to produce a bottle of water. Additionally, think of the cost of wrapping, transporting, cooling, collecting and recycling all of those bottles is money that could be spent on other things to enhance our communities if the industry didn't exist on such a massive scale.

In the United States, we consume about thirty billion water bottles every year. Of the fifty billion water bottles drunk worldwide, the US consumption is about sixty percent of the entire world's usage even though we are only a fraction over four percent of the world's population.

The year 2011 holds the record for the high point in regards to bottled water sales. 9.1 billion gallons were sold. This was an historical record. The Earth Policy Institute estimates the resources needed just to transport, store and sell the bottled water exceeds fifty million barrels of oil and a fleet of over forty thousand trucks just to deliver. This estimate includes the delivery of exotic waters such as Fiji, San Pellegrino and even Perrier. These are huge amounts of wasted resources when all you need to do is turn on a tap.

The type of plastic used to manufacture water bottles is called PET plastics. They don't biodegrade like food particles do, rather they photodegrade. That means they break down into smaller and smaller bits over time. These bits get into our waterways, contaminate our soil and sicken animals when they eat plastic, thinking it might be food. Many dead whales, birds and other animals have been found with stomachs full of plastic bits instead of real food the animals needed to survive.

The Ocean Conservancy say the most common pollutant found in the ocean, on the ocean floor and on our beaches is plastic. This plastic will never degrade, but only break down into smaller and smaller bits, eventually settling onto the ocean floor.

Grab a glass and turn on a faucet to satisfy your thirst and save the environment. If your water is not great, get a reverse osmosis or other filtration system so it is good water. The cost will pay you back in great health dividends and think of how much you will save by not buying bottled water.

Cities throughout the world are banning plastic water bottles just as they are reducing or eliminating plastic shopping bags. In Australia, the town of Bundanoon in New South Wales voted to totally ban the use and sale of plastic water bottles. They have made filtered refilling stations, drinking fountains available instead.

The Grand Canyon National Park approved a plan to ban plastic water bottles and have also made drinking and water stations available throughout the park. Many zoos don't have straws or cups with lids because people would through them into the water with the animals. Disney Parks and Universal will give you a cup to fill from the many water fountains around the parks. These parks have been known for taking bottled water from patrons as they enter.

What can you do?

- Use a refillable, non-plastic, water bottle. Avoid BPA plastics, look for the BPA-Free label
- Check the quality of your tap water; get a filter if it makes you feel better. We have reverse osmosis on our house water.
- Do the research! Don't fall for marketing ploys that tell you bottled water is good. They are selling a product and the goal is profit. They have no concern for your personal health.
- Recycle effectively so your waste actually does get recycled.

What if you don't like the way the tap water tastes?

Filter it. You can get Brita filters to do a pitcher or a couple of gallons. If you are traveling, you will discover the water will have different flavors at different locations. Well water is different and can be fresh, bright and clean, or strong and pungent with sulfur as found in the midsection of Florida. Water from Yosemite National Park has some of the purest water and is the water source for San Francisco. The water from Yosemite is so pure, filtration is not necessary.

Did you know…?

New York City has the safest, cleanest water in the entire country?

You are throwing your money away when you buy bottled water.

To compare the cost of bottled water to tap water: If you were to use only bottled water for your household, washing dishes, showers, watering plants, your monthly bill would be in the range of $9,000.

Bottled water costs over 1,000 times more than tap, even filtered tap water. Ditch the plastic bottles!

If you care about the human impact on the planet, we can make a difference today by choosing to use refillable drink bottles.

Make a statement with your water bottle, *own it*, make it chic to carry a refillable bottle.

I carry *Contigo* water bottles. This company makes quite a variety and the best part is they don't leak. They can keep drinks cold, chilled, or warm. They are not thermal but are insulated by a double wall of stainless.

I take one with me everywhere and I have discovered refilling stations easily every time I have needed one.

PART II

Healthy & Hydrated

The Next Step:

Taking Care of Your Skin

Outside In

13. HYDRATING FROM THE OUTSIDE IN

Hydrating your skin from the outside is one of the secrets to a youthful glow.

As you age, the skin thins and can become delicate. Using skin nourishing products on your skin can help keep the skin strong and prevent the "old people bruising" and crepe paper skin that is so common on older people's arms and legs.

Well hydrated skin helps prevent disease by protecting the body from the outside world. Dry, damaged skin leaves room for infection to invade and cause issues of all kinds.

We know that some chemicals can and do enter your bloodstream through topical application.

The task of scrutinizing every ingredient in the bevy of daily products the average family uses can be daunting. Instead of tackling the entire project at once, break it down into more manageable pieces.

Start with the products that are having the most negative impact. There is a list of some product ideas to get you started on the next page.

Different products mean different levels of exposure and concern. For instance, if you use a lotion all over your body; it soaks into your skin all day. That's more exposure to those chemicals than if you were to use the same ingredients in a face cleanser that is washed off.

Shampoo and conditioner wash over your body when used. It's not just getting on your hair, but runs down your back, face, sometimes into your eyes, ears and mouth.

You can be strategic.

Get the best ingredients in products that you have a lot of exposure to like shampoo, lotion, bath soaks, or sunscreen. Then, if you want to, relax your standards a bit for products like hand soap, however, a good organic hand soap is easy to find these days.

YOU DON'T HAVE TO BE PERFECT!

When you try to be perfect it can be overwhelming and then we get paralyzed. Sometimes we just want to buy something and trust that it is good for us and won't cause any harm.

The way to avoid being overwhelmed is by choosing when to demand a certain standard and when it's ok to relax that standard a little bit. That way you don't have to worry about every ingredient all the time and you can still drastically improve the overall quality of your beauty and skin care products.

Find a company you trust. Some of the best beauty products are hand crafted in small batches using natural and organic herbs, spices, oils, and butters by artisans rather than by giant companies that sell products worldwide.

Top products to look for cleanest ingredients:

➤ Anything you soak in such as bubble bath, or bath salts for soaking

Anything you apply and do not wash off, such as lotion, face and body creams, and oils

➤ Body powder – careful of particle inhalation

➤ Shampoo and conditioner are wash-off products but have high exposure due to how the product is used. Consider the way shampoos and conditioners spill over your face and entire body; into your mouth, eyes, ears and nose as you wash and rinse your hair.

➤ Any product you put on your child. They are so young and have such tender systems. It doesn't take much.

7 Questionable Ingredients to Avoid

Certain chemical ingredients can potentially cause problems for your skin when applied as a liquid or bar soap and are best avoided.

Sodium Lauryl/Laureth Sulfate (SLS/SLES)

Sodium lauryl sulfate is a surfactant, detergent, and emulsifier used in thousands of cosmetic products, as well as in industrial cleaners. Present in nearly all shampoos, toothpastes, body washes, and cleansers, liquid hand soaps, laundry detergents, and bath oils and bath salts.

Although SLS originates from coconuts, the manufacturing process results in SLES/SLS being contaminated with 1,4 dioxane, a carcinogenic byproduct.

SLS is the sodium salt of lauryl sulfate, and is rated by the Environmental Working Group's (EWG) Skin Deep Cosmetics Database as a "moderate hazard."

SLS breaks down the skin's moisture barrier, easily penetrates the skin, and allows other chemicals to penetrate by increasing skin permeability by approximately 100-fold.

Combined with other chemicals, SLS becomes a "nitrosamine," a potent class of carcinogen.

Research studies have linked SLS to skin and eye irritation, organ toxicity, reproductive and developmental toxicity and endocrine disruption.

Dioxane

Dioxane is common in a wide range of products as part of PEG, Polysorbates, Laureth, and ethoxylated alcohols. These compounds are usually contaminated with high concentrations of highly volatile 1,4-dioxane which is easily absorbed through the skin.

This "probable carcinogen to humans" substance has received a "high hazard" rating from EWG's Skin Deep and is especially toxic to your brain, central nervous system, kidneys, and liver.

A synthetic derivative of coconut, watch for misleading language on labels, stating "comes from coconut."

Avoid any product with indications of ethoxylation, which include: "myreth," "oleth," "laureth," "ceteareth," any other "eth," "PEG," "polyethylene," "polyethylene glycol," "polyoxyethylene," or "oxynol," in ingredient names.

Parabens

Parabens are widely used as preservatives in an estimated 13,200 cosmetic and skin care products.

Parabens have hormone-disrupting qualities, mimicking estrogen, and interfere with the body's endocrine system. Studies have shown that parabens can affect your body much like estrogens, which can lead to diminished muscle mass, extra fat storage, and male breast growth.

The EPA has linked methyl parabens, in particular, to metabolic, developmental, hormonal, and neurological disorders.

Propylene Glycol

Propylene glycol a common ingredient in personal care products, it's been shown to cause dermatitis, kidney or liver abnormalities, and may inhibit skin cell growth or cause skin irritation.

Also found in engine coolants, antifreeze, rubber cleaners, adhesives, and paints and varnishes.

Diethanolamine or DEA

DEA readily reacts with nitrite preservatives and contaminants to create nitrosodiethanolamine (NDEA), a known and potent carcinogen.

DEA also appears to block absorption of the nutrient choline, vital to brain development.

Fragrance

Toluene, made from petroleum or coal tar, is found in most synthetic fragrances. Chronic exposure is linked to anemia, lowered blood cell count, liver or kidney damage, and may affect a developing fetus.

Synthetic fragrances can also be drying and irritating to your skin.

Fragrance is the new second hand smoke.

Triclosan

Triclosan is the antibacterial agent added to many liquid hand soaps to help kill germs. Triclosan is suspected of contributing to the growing problem of antibiotic resistance.

There are communities with septic systems that ban the use of products that contain Triclosan because of how they destroy the biological patterns of a proper working septic tank.

Triclosan destroys the natural lipid balance of your skin making it more susceptible to damage and dryness.

Recent research has shown that home spa treatments are now a billion dollar industry. People are taking better care of their skin and are learning about ingredients to avoid and which ingredients to use to promote skin health.

People are learning how to use specialized products at home so routine facials and body scrubs are more common than the occasional spa visit. With daily schedules as full and robust as they are, being able to take great care of our skin and create an at home spa experience is one key to sanity.

The skin is the largest organ of the body. Its function is vital. Skin covers our entire body and is made up of 64% water.

To illustrate hydration and the effects of dehydration on the body, think of how fresh fruit shrivels as it dries out. That is what happens to your skin. Keeping it hydrated helps it stay youthfully lifted and fills out those wrinkles and fine lines.

This book means to increase awareness of how important the simple act of drinking water is to the proper functioning of the human body. While the body does operate in various states of dehydration all of the time, to maintain a high level of health and good quality of life, hydration is critical.

I challenge you to measure your hydration intake vs. your daily need.

Try it for three weeks and make note of the differences you feel.

1. **Are you meeting your daily hydration needs?**

2. **How do you want to live out your life and golden years? How do you want to age?**

3. **The choice is yours, what action will you take?**

If you suffer from heart disease or are under care for your heart for any reason, you will need to consult your doctor for advice and approval to begin a water consumption routine. With many kinds of heart disease, fluids are restricted. Always get your cardiologists approval if under medical care.

Additionally, if you are taking medications or have any dietary restrictions, ALWAYS consult your doctor and medical care team before starting or changing any current regime you are on. This includes increasing your water intake.

This advice is intended for normal, healthy individuals who live active lifestyles and have no serious medical issues.

This advice is not intended to replace, supersede or discount any medical professionals care plan. If you have questions, consult your medical care team for personalized advisement.

14. APPENDIX:

1. Links to tomato research

2. Environmental Working Group (EWG): The Dirty Dozen

3. EWG: Clean 15

4. Chart of High Hydrating Foods

5. FAQ

Studies supporting tomato nutrient research:

http://www.hort.purdue.edu/ext/HO-26.PDF

http://ndb.nal.usda.gov/ndb/foods/show/3258

http://www.fao.org/fileadmin/templates/agns/pdf/jecfa/cta/71/lycopene_extract_from_tomato.pdf

Studies supporting bottled water impact

http://pacinst.org/publication/bottled-water-and-energy-a-fact-sheet/

http://www.huffingtonpost.com/normschriever/post_5218_b_3613577.html

EWG Dirty Dozen

The items on this list represent the product that research testing has discovered large amounts of pesticides. These are the items you should always buy organic.

1. Strawberries
2. Apples
3. Nectarines
4. Peaches
5. Celery
6. Grapes
7. Cherries
8. Spinach
9. Tomatoes
10. Bell Peppers
11. Cherry Tomatoes
12. Cucumbers

EWG Clean 15

The items on this list are where you can be more lenient. However, be on the lookout for GMO foods. If you buy organic, you avoid GMO's.

1. Avocados
2. Corn
3. Pineapples
4. Cabbage
5. Sweet Peas
6. Onions
7. Asparagus
8. Mangoes
9. Papaya
10. Kiwi
11. Eggplant
12. Honeydew
13. Grapefruit
14. Cantaloupe
15. Cauliflower

Contact **The Environmental Working Group** *at www.ewg.org for more information.*

High Hydrating Foods — Above 90% Water

Cucumber	96.7%
Iceberg Lettuce	95.6%
Celery	95.4%
Radishes	95.3%
Tomatoes	94.5%
Green Peppers	93.9%
Red or yellow peppers	92%
Cauliflower	92.1%
Watermelon	91.5%
Spinach	91.4%
Star Fruit	91.4%
Strawberries	91%
Broccoli	90.7%
Grapefruit	90.5%
Baby Carrots	90.4%
Cantaloupe	90.2%

15. FREQUENTLY ASKED QUESTIONS

I'm a vegan and I get really tired in the afternoons. It's a real energy drain and I need to take a nap. How can I get over this afternoon slump?

Try eating some high protein and high hydration snacks right after lunch. Celery with nut butters, protein bars with a glass of water, Broccoli has the highest protein of all the vegetables so dip broccoli into hummus. Your body needs a source of energy and so give it something to work with. Make sure your water intake levels are steady throughout the day. Dehydration is the #1 cause of daytime fatigue.

I really don't like the taste of water. What do you suggest?

Try flavoring your water with citrus, fruits or herbal teas. Cucumber, carrot, watermelon, cantaloupe and other melons, berries all add very nice natural flavors to water without adding extra sugar. It is essential you find something you can drink daily. Your good health depends upon it. Ultimately, the choice is yours; I hope you select good health.

If I drink all that water, won't I be peeing all day?

Yes, you will eliminate whatever water your body does not use, taking toxins and other bodily wastes with it. The less time toxins stay in your body, the fewer problems they can cause. Your urine should be a very pale yellow or near colorless. If it is dark, you need to be drinking some water over the next few hours, please, not all at once.

Healthy & Hydrated is affiliated with Lotions & Potions, All Natural Skin Care. Your skin care completes the cycle of hydration from the *Inside Out and the Outside In.*

Lotions & Potions All Natural Skin Care is a small artisan company that handcrafts high quality, natural skin care products in Charlotte, NC

Visit the online store by visiting

www.chefpamelafoodhealthandwellness.com/shoponline

Or by scanning this QR Code

Subscription and custom services available. Please use the mail below.

Send wholesale inquiries to:

info@chefpamela.com

16. ABOUT THE AUTHOR

Pamela Roberts is a Certified Executive Chef and Certified Culinary Educator through the American Culinary Federation.

She is the host of her own cooking show named *Charlotte Cooks,* on PBS-Charlotte. *Charlotte Cooks* can be viewed on You Tube for those out of the regional PBS area.

Pamela has been passionate about food since a young age, believing in a direct connection between food and health.

Pamela studies and practices herbalism, aromatherapy, mindset theories and nutrition. Her mission with this book is to inspire others to increase the amount of water they drink thereby improving their health and the way they age.

Pamela believes that once people understand why and how, it is easy to then make decisions that makes the best sense to each person.

Pamela lives and teaches culinary school in Charlotte, North Carolina. She is a professional speaker and presenter teaching seminars and workshops to businesses, groups and individuals who want to learn more about how to increase their health through hydration and the foods they eat and natural skin care.

For more information, send an e mail to:

info@chefpamela.com

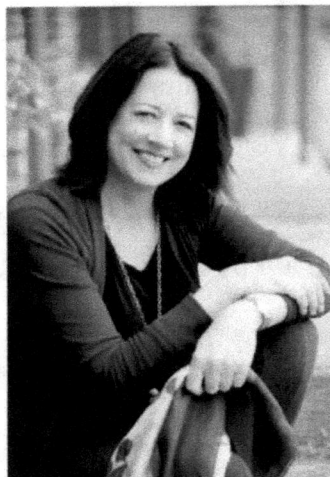

www.ingramcontent.com/pod-product-compliance
Lightning Source LLC
Chambersburg PA
CBHW050543280326
41933CB00011B/1699